SCHIZOPHRENIA DIET PLAN COOK BOOK

A Schizophrenia Diet Plan for Making Healthy Food Choices That Aid Cognitive Function

REX LEWIS

Table of Contents

B

Introduction

Schizophrenia Is A Multifaceted Psychiatric Condition Marked By A Variety Of Symptoms, Such As Hallucinations, Delusions, Disordered Thinking, And Reduced Cognitive Abilities. Although There Is No Single Diet That May Cure Or Treat Schizophrenia, Certain Studies Indicate That Nutrition May Contribute To The Overall Mental Health And Well-Being Of Individuals With This Disorder.

It Is Crucial To Acknowledge That A Nutritious Diet Is Advantageous For All Individuals, Irrespective Of Their Mental Health Status. Nevertheless, Individuals Diagnosed With

Schizophrenia May Encounter Distinctive Obstacles Concerning Their Medicine, Way Of Life, And The Possibility Of Weight Increase Linked To Specific Antipsychotic Medications.

Several Overarching Dietary Guidelines For Patients With Schizophrenia Include:

• Prioritize A Nutritionally Balanced Diet That Encompasses A Diverse Range Of Fruits, Vegetables, Whole Grains, Lean Meats, And Beneficial Fats. An Alimentary Regimen That Is Rich In Nutrients Can Positively Impact Both The Physical And Mental State Of An Individual.

• Omega-3 Fatty Acids, Which May Be Found In Fatty Fish Like Salmon And Trout, As Well As In Flaxseeds And Walnuts, Have Been Linked To Potential Mental Health Advantages According To Certain Research. Omega-3 Fatty Acids Have A Crucial Role In Brain Function And Possess Potential Anti-Inflammatory Qualities.

• Sufficient Consumption Of Vital Vitamins And Minerals, Including Vitamin D, B-Vitamins, Zinc, And Magnesium, Is Crucial For Maintaining Good Health. Insufficiencies In These Essential Nutrients Can Have An Adverse Effect On Mental Well-Being.

• Restricting The Consumption Of Sugar And Processed Foods: Diets

That Are Abundant In Sugar And Processed Foods Have The Potential To Promote Inflammation And Have Adverse Effects On Mental Well-Being. It Is Generally Advised To Follow A Diet That Mostly Consists Of Whole, Nutrient-Rich Foods.

• Evaluation Of Adverse Effects Of Medication: Certain Antipsychotic Drugs Have The Potential To Cause Weight Gain And Metabolic Complications. Collaborating With A Healthcare Practitioner Or A Qualified Dietitian Can Assist In Weight Management And Handle Potential Side Effects By Making Informed Food Decisions.

Collaboration Between Individuals With Schizophrenia And Healthcare Specialists, Such As Psychiatrists, Psychologists, And Nutritionists, Is Essential In Developing A Thorough Treatment Plan That Caters To Their Specific Requirements. Nutrition Can Complement Conventional Medical Treatment In Controlling Schizophrenia, But It Should Not Be Considered A Replacement For Medication And Therapy. It Is Always Advisable To Seek Guidance From Healthcare Professionals Who Can Provide Specialized Counsel Tailored To Your Specific Health Needs And Circumstances.

CHAPTER ONE
The Connection between Diet and Schizophrenia

The Connection Between Diet And Schizophrenia Is An Area Of Ongoing Research, And While No Specific Dietary Interventions Can Replace Traditional Treatments, There Is Evidence To Suggest That Nutrition May Play A Role In Supporting Mental Health For Individuals With Schizophrenia. Here Are Some Aspects Of The Connection Between Diet And Schizophrenia:

• **Nutrient Deficiencies:** Some Studies Have Indicated That Individuals With Schizophrenia May Be At A Higher Risk Of Certain Nutrient Deficiencies,

Such As Low Levels Of Vitamin D, B-Vitamins, And Essential Minerals Like Zinc And Magnesium. These Nutrients Are Crucial For Brain Function, And Their Deficiency May Impact Mental Health.

• **Inflammation:** Inflammation Has Been Linked To Various Mental Health Conditions, Including Schizophrenia. Diets High In Processed Foods, Sugars, And Saturated Fats May Contribute To Inflammation, While Diets Rich In Fruits, Vegetables, And Omega-3 Fatty Acids May Have Anti-Inflammatory Effects.

• **Omega-3 Fatty Acids:** Research Has Suggested That Omega-3 Fatty Acids, Particularly EPA And DHA Found In

Fatty Fish, May Have Potential Benefits For Individuals With Schizophrenia. Omega-3s Are Essential For Brain Function, And Some Studies Have Explored Their Role In Reducing Symptoms And Improving Cognitive Function In Schizophrenia Patients.

• **Gluten And Casein Sensitivity:** Some Individuals With Schizophrenia May Have Sensitivities To Gluten (Found In Wheat) And Casein (Found In Dairy). While This Is Not A Universal Phenomenon, Some Studies Have Explored The Impact Of Gluten-Free And Casein-Free Diets On Symptom Improvement For Certain Individuals With Schizophrenia.

• **Weight Gain And Medication Side Effects:** Many Individuals With Schizophrenia Take Antipsychotic Medications That Can Lead To Weight Gain And Metabolic Issues. Managing Weight Through A Balanced Diet And Regular Exercise Is Important For Overall Health And May Help Mitigate Some Medication-Related Side Effects.

It's Essential To Approach Dietary Interventions With Caution And Under The Guidance Of Healthcare Professionals. Each Person With Schizophrenia May Have Unique Nutritional Needs And Responses To Specific Dietary Changes. Consulting With A Registered Dietitian Or Nutritionist, In Collaboration With

Mental Health Professionals, Can Help Develop An Individualized Plan That Considers Both Physical And Mental Health Aspects.

While Nutritional Interventions Can Play A Supportive Role, They Are Not A Substitute For Prescribed Medications And Other Evidence-Based Treatments For Schizophrenia. Anyone With Schizophrenia Or Concerned About Their Mental Health Should Seek Guidance From A Qualified Healthcare Professional For A Comprehensive And Personalized Approach To Care.

Foundations of a Schizophrenia-Friendly Diet

Nutritionally Packed Foods That Promote General Health And Wellness Are The Foundation Of A Schizophrenia-Friendly Diet. Although There Isn't A Silver Bullet, People Living With Schizophrenia Can Benefit From The Following Principles:

Balanced Diet:

• Emphasize A Variety Of Whole Foods, Including Fruits, Vegetables, Whole Grains, Lean Proteins, And Healthy Fats.

• Strive For Balance In Macronutrients (Carbohydrates, Proteins, And Fats)

To Provide A Steady And Sustained Source Of Energy.

Omega-3 Fatty Acids:

• Incorporate Sources Of Omega-3 Fatty Acids, Such As Fatty Fish (Salmon, Mackerel), Flaxseeds, Chia Seeds, And Walnuts. Omega-3s Are Essential For Brain Health And May Have Anti-Inflammatory Properties.

Vitamins And Minerals:

• Ensure Adequate Intake Of Essential Nutrients, Including Vitamin D, B-Vitamins (Especially Folate And B12), Zinc, And Magnesium. These Nutrients Play A Role In Cognitive Function And Overall Mental Health.

Low-Glycemic Foods:

• Choose Complex Carbohydrates With A Low Glycemic Index To Help Maintain Stable Blood Sugar Levels. This Includes Whole Grains, Legumes, And Non-Starchy Vegetables.

Protein Sources:

• Include Lean Protein Sources Such As Poultry, Fish, Tofu, Legumes, And Nuts. Protein Is Essential For Neurotransmitter Synthesis And Overall Cellular Function.

Limit Sugar And Processed Foods:

• Minimize The Consumption Of Sugary Foods And Beverages, As Well As Processed And Refined Foods. Diets High In Sugar And Processed Foods

May Contribute To Inflammation And Negatively Impact Mental Health.

Hydration:

• Stay Adequately Hydrated By Drinking Water Throughout The Day. Dehydration Can Impact Cognitive Function And Overall Well-Being.

Consider Individual Sensitivities:

• Some Individuals With Schizophrenia May Have Sensitivities To Gluten Or Casein. If There Is Suspicion Of Such Sensitivities, Working With A Healthcare Professional To Explore A Gluten-Free Or Casein-Free Diet May Be Considered.

Meal Regularity:

• Aim For Regular Meal Times To Provide A Consistent Source Of Energy Throughout The Day. Irregular Eating Patterns May Contribute To Fluctuations In Blood Sugar Levels.

Collaboration With Healthcare Professionals:

• Work Closely With Healthcare Professionals, Including Psychiatrists, Psychologists, And Dietitians, To Develop A Comprehensive Treatment Plan. Nutritional Considerations Should Be Integrated Into The Overall Care Plan.

It's Important To Note That These Guidelines Are General

Recommendations, And Individual Variations Exist. The Key Is To Tailor The Diet To The Specific Needs And Preferences Of The Individual With Schizophrenia. Regular Monitoring And Adjustment, In Collaboration With Healthcare Professionals, Can Help Optimize The Nutritional Approach As Part Of A Comprehensive Treatment Plan For Schizophrenia.

CHAPTER TWO
Specific Nutrients for Schizophrenia Management

Several Nutrients Play A Role In Brain Health, And Their Intake May Be Particularly Relevant For Individuals With Schizophrenia. While Nutritional Needs Can Vary Among Individuals, Here Are Some Specific Nutrients That Have Been Studied In The Context Of Schizophrenia Management:

Omega-3 Fatty Acids:

- **Source:** Fatty Fish (Salmon, Mackerel, Trout), Flaxseeds, Chia Seeds, Walnuts.

- **Role:** Omega-3s, Particularly EPA (Eicosapentaenoic Acid) And DHA (Docosahexaenoic

Acid), Are Crucial For Brain Function. Some Studies Suggest That Omega-3 Supplementation May Help Reduce Symptoms And Improve Cognitive Function In Individuals With Schizophrenia.

Vitamin D:

- **Source:** Sunlight Exposure, Fatty Fish, Fortified Dairy Products, And Supplements If Needed.

- **Role:** Vitamin D Is Essential For Overall Health, Including Brain Health. Some Studies Have Found Associations Between Low Vitamin D Levels And

Increased Risk Of Schizophrenia.

B-Vitamins:

- **Sources:** Whole Grains, Meat, Poultry, Fish, Eggs, Dairy Products, Leafy Greens.

- **Role:** B-Vitamins, Including Folate (B9) And B12, Are Involved In Neurotransmitter Synthesis And Play A Role In Cognitive Function. Deficiencies In These Vitamins Have Been Associated With Schizophrenia.

Zinc:

- **Sources:** Meat, Poultry, Seafood, Nuts, Seeds, And Legumes.

- **Role:** Zinc Is Involved In Various Cellular Processes, And Some Studies Suggest That Individuals With Schizophrenia May Have Lower Zinc Levels. Adequate Zinc Intake Is Important For Overall Mental Health.

Magnesium:

- **Sources:** Nuts, Seeds, Whole Grains, Leafy Green Vegetables.
- **Role:** Magnesium Is Involved In Neurotransmitter Function And May Have A Role In Supporting Mental Health. Some Research Has Explored Magnesium Supplementation As A Potential

Adjunctive Treatment For Schizophrenia.

Antioxidants:

- **Sources:** Fruits And Vegetables (Especially Berries, Citrus Fruits, And Leafy Greens).

- **Role:** Antioxidants Help Combat Oxidative Stress, Which May Be Elevated In Individuals With Schizophrenia. A Diet Rich In Fruits And Vegetables Provides A Range Of Antioxidants.

Protein:

- **Sources:** Lean Meats, Poultry, Fish, Tofu, Legumes, Nuts, And Seeds.

- **Role:** Proteins Are Essential For Neurotransmitter Synthesis And Overall Cellular Function. Adequate Protein Intake Is Important For Maintaining Overall Health.

Taurine:

- **Sources:** Meat, Fish, Dairy Products.
- **Role:** Taurine Is An Amino Acid That Plays A Role In Neurotransmitter Regulation. Some Studies Have Investigated The Potential Benefits Of Taurine Supplementation In Individuals With Schizophrenia.

It's Crucial To Approach Nutritional Interventions With Guidance From Healthcare Professionals, As Individual Needs And Responses Can Vary. Nutrient Supplementation Should Be Tailored To Individual Requirements And Should Not Replace Prescribed Medications Or Other Evidence-Based Treatments For Schizophrenia. Working Collaboratively With Healthcare Providers, Including Psychiatrists And Dietitians, Ensures A Comprehensive And Personalized Approach To Managing Schizophrenia Through Nutrition.

Foods to Include and Avoid

While There Is No Specific "Schizophrenia Diet," Incorporating A Balanced And Nutrient-Dense Approach To Eating Can Be Beneficial For Individuals With Schizophrenia. Here Are Some General Guidelines For Foods To Include And Avoid:

Foods To Include:

• **Fruits and Vegetables:** Include A Variety Of Colorful Fruits And Vegetables. They Provide Essential Vitamins, Minerals, And Antioxidants.

• **Whole Grains:** Opt For Whole Grains Such As Brown Rice, Quinoa, Oats, And Whole Wheat. These Provide Complex Carbohydrates For Sustained Energy.

• **Lean Proteins:** Choose Lean Sources Of Protein, Including Poultry, Fish, Tofu, Legumes, Nuts, And Seeds. Protein Is Important For Neurotransmitter Synthesis.

• **Fatty Fish:** Incorporate Fatty Fish Like Salmon, Mackerel, And Trout For Omega-3 Fatty Acids, Which Are Beneficial For Brain Health.

• **Nuts and Seeds:** Include Nuts And Seeds, Such As Walnuts, Flaxseeds, And Chia Seeds, For Healthy Fats And Essential Nutrients.

• **Dairy Or Dairy Alternatives:** Consume Dairy Products Or Fortified Alternatives For Calcium And Vitamin D, Important For Bone Health.

- **Hydration:** Drink Plenty Of Water Throughout The Day To Stay Hydrated. Dehydration Can Affect Cognitive Function.

- **Herbs And Spices:** Use Herbs And Spices To Add Flavor To Meals. Some, Like Turmeric, May Have Anti-Inflammatory Properties.

Foods To Limit Or Avoid:

- **Processed and Sugary Foods:** Limit Intake Of Processed Foods, Sugary Snacks, And Beverages. These Can Contribute To Inflammation And May Negatively Impact Mental Health.

- **Highly Processed Meats:** Reduce Consumption Of Highly Processed Meats, Such As Sausages And Deli

Meats. Opt For Leaner, Unprocessed Protein Sources.

• **Excessive Caffeine:** Moderate Caffeine Intake, As Excessive Amounts May Contribute To Anxiety And Disrupt Sleep Patterns.

• **Alcohol:** Limit Alcohol Consumption, As It Can Interact With Medications And Affect Mental Health.

• **High-Fat And Fried Foods:** Limit The Intake Of High-Fat And Fried Foods, As They May Contribute To Weight Gain And Overall Health Issues.

Gluten And Casein (If Sensitive): Some Individuals With Schizophrenia May Have Sensitivities To Gluten

(Found In Wheat) Or Casein (Found In Dairy). If There Are Suspicions Of Sensitivities, Consultation With A Healthcare Professional May Be Necessary.

• **Artificial Additives:** Minimize The Consumption Of Artificial Additives, Preservatives, And Artificial Sweeteners.

It's Important To Note That Individual Responses To Specific Foods Can Vary, And Any Dietary Changes Should Be Discussed With Healthcare Professionals. Additionally, Nutritional Needs Can Be Influenced By Factors Such As Medication Side Effects, Comorbid Health Conditions, And Lifestyle Factors. A Personalized

Approach, With Input From Healthcare Providers And, If Possible, A Registered Dietitian, Is Essential For Creating A Diet That Supports Both Physical And Mental Well-Being In Individuals With Schizophrenia.

CHAPTER THREE
Strategies for Eating Well For People Living With Schizophrenia

Developing A Healthy, Well-Rounded Diet Is An Important Part Of Meal Planning For People With Schizophrenia. Some Broad Principles For Meal Preparation Are As Follows:

1. Stick To A Regular Meal Schedule: Make Sure You Eat At The Same Times Every Day So You Have A Steady Supply Of Energy. Substitute Snacks For One Or More Of Your Main Meals.

2. Macronutrient Balance: Keep The Carbs, Proteins, And Fats In Your Meals At A Reasonable Ratio. This Aids In Providing Steady Energy And

Bolsters A Number Of Physiological Processes.

3. Eat Your Veggies And Fruits: Make Sure To Include A Rainbow Of Colorful Fruits And Veggies With Every Meal. Their Vitamin, Mineral, And Antioxidant Content Is Vital.

4. Whole Grains: Pick Out Whole Grains Like Quinoa, Brown Rice, Oats, And Wheat. You Can Get Long-Lasting Energy From These Complex Carbs.

5. Lean Proteins: Make Sure To Incorporate Lean Protein Sources Into Your Diet, Such As Lean Meats, Fish, Tofu, Beans, Seeds, And Nuts. When Making Neurotransmitters, Protein Plays A Crucial Role.

6. Omega-3 Fatty Acids From Fatty Fish: Include Fatty Fish In Your Diet, Such As Salmon, Mackerel, Or Trout, To Supply Your Brain With Omega-3 Fatty Acids.

7. Nuts And Seeds: Consume Walnuts, Flaxseeds, Or Chia Seeds As A Snack To Provide Extra Nutrients And Healthy Fats To Your Diet.

8. Eighth, Dairy Or Dairy Substitutes: OGive Your Bones The Calcium And Vitamin D They Need By Eating Dairy Products Or Fortified Dairy Substitutes.

9. Make Sure You Drink Enough Water Throughout The Day To Stay Properly

Hydrated. 9. Cognitive Function Can Be Affected By Dehydration.

10. Cut Back On Sugar And Processed Foods: Eat Less Sugary Snacks And Processed Foods. Instead, Go For Full, Nutrient-Dense Foods.

11. Moderation with Caffeine: Limit Your Caffeine Use; Too Much Of It Can Make You Anxious And Make It Hard To Sleep.

12. Practice Mindful Eating: Teach People To Pay Attention To Their Bodies By Observing Signals For When They Are Hungry Or Full. For A More Satisfying Meal, Try Not To Multitask.

13. Take Medications Into Account: O Think About When You Eat In Relation

To When You Take Your Medicine, If That's Relevant. Consult Your Healthcare Provider For Advice On Whether To Take Your Medication With Or Without Food.

14. Personal Preferences And Intolerances: Think About People's Specific Dietary Needs, Food Allergies, And Dietary Limitations.

15. Talk To Your Doctor: It's A Good Idea To Talk To Your Doctor, Psychiatrist, Or Nutritionist On A Regular Basis About Your Health, Any Changes In Your Diet, And Any Adverse Affects Of Your Medications.

Personalizing Diet Programs To Meet Dietary Restrictions And Personal

Tastes Is Essential. An Individual's Specific Needs, Such As Food Allergies Or Drug Interactions, Can Be Better Met With The Individualized Attention Of A Nutritionist Or Registered Dietitian. Creating A Welcoming And Supportive Dining Space And Include The Person In Meal Planning Are Two More Factors That Can Improve Health.

Integrating Dietary Modifications Into One's Lifestyle

Integrating Dietary Modifications Into One's Daily Routine, Particularly For Persons Who Are Treating Schizophrenia, Can Be A Progressive And Beneficial Endeavor. Here Are Some Pragmatic Suggestions To

Facilitate The Incorporation Of Dietary Modifications Into One's Everyday Routine:

• **Commence Gradually:** Initiate With Minor, Feasible Alterations To Prevent Experiencing A Sense Of Being Overwhelmed. This Could Involve Integrating A Single Nutritious Food Item Or Making Incremental Changes To One Meal At A Time.

• Establish Attainable And Pragmatic Dietary Objectives By Setting Realistic Targets. This May Entail Augmenting The Consumption Of Fruits And Vegetables, Opting For Healthy Grains, Or Integrating Additional Sources Of Lean Protein.

• **Meal Prepping:** Plan And Organize Meals Ahead Of Time To Ensure Convenient Access To Healthier Food Choices. Preparing Nutritious Meals In Advance Can Reduce The Need To Depend On Easy Yet Less Nutritious Alternatives.

• **Discover New Recipes**: Engage In Culinary Experimentation By Trying Out Novel Recipes That Incorporate A Diverse Range Of Foods Rich In Nutrients. This Can Enhance The Excitement Of The Diet And Make The Changeover More Pleasurable.

• **Enhance Knowledge And Engage:** Acquire Knowledge For Yourself And Individuals Involved In Meal Preparation Regarding The

Advantages Of Particular Meals For Mental Well-Being. Engaging Family Or Friends In The Process Helps Foster A Nurturing Environment.

• Engage In Mindful Eating By Attentively Observing Hunger And Satiety Signals. This Entails Relishing Every Mouthful And Maintaining Mindfulness During Meals.

• Establish A Hydration Regimen By Consuming Water Consistently Throughout The Day. Utilize A Reusable Water Bottle As A Prompt To Maintain Proper Hydration.

• **Obtain Expert Assistance:** Engage The Services Of A Certified Dietitian Or Nutritionist To Acquire Tailored

Recommendations And Direction That Align With Specific Requirements, Preferences, And Health Circumstances.

• **Manage Food Sensitivities:** If There Are Concerns With Gluten, Dairy, Or Other Food Sensitivities, Collaborate With Healthcare Specialists To Identify And Resolve Any Potential Problems.

• **Social Support:** Participate In Social Events That Promote The Selection Of Healthier Dietary Options. Having A Network Of Supportive Friends And Family Can Enhance The Experience Of Transitioning To A New Diet.

• **Establish A Conducive Eating Environment:** Cultivate A Positive

And Tranquil Atmosphere For Meals. Minimize The Presence Of Electronic Devices, Such As Screens, At Mealtime And Direct Your Attention On Fully Savoring The Dining Experience.

• **Maintain Adaptability:** Remain Flexible And Receptive To Modifications. Striking A Harmonious Equilibrium Between Health Objectives And Personal Preferences Is Crucial For Maintaining Lasting Transformations.

• Recognize And Commemorate Accomplishments, Regardless Of Their Magnitude. Positive Reinforcement Is Effective In Motivating Sustained Efforts.

• **Comprehend Medicine Interactions:** Take Into Account The Time Of Meals In Relation To Medicine, And Collaborate With Healthcare Providers To Ensure That Dietary Modifications Are In Line With Drug Administration.

• Continuously Monitor And Evaluate The Progress, And Be Prepared To Make Necessary Adjustments. One's Dietary Requirements May Change Over Time, And It Is Crucial To Continuously Assess And Monitor Them.

It Is Important To Keep In Mind That Embracing A More Healthful Way Of Life Is A Process, And Obstacles May Arise. It Is Crucial To Adopt A Positive

Mindset And Perceive Dietary Changes As An Integral Component Of A Comprehensive Approach To General Well-Being. Seeking Guidance From Medical Experts And Engaging With A Strong Support System Can Enhance The Effectiveness Of Integrating Dietary Modifications Into The Daily Routine Of Those Coping With Schizophrenia.

CHAPTER FOUR
Types Of Physical Activities For Mental Health

Engaging In Regular Physical Activity Is Not Only Beneficial For Physical Health But Also Plays A Crucial Role In Promoting Mental Well-Being. Various Types Of Physical Activities Can Positively Impact Mental Health By Reducing Stress, Improving Mood, Enhancing Cognitive Function, And Alleviating Symptoms Of Conditions Like Anxiety And Depression. Here Are Different Types Of Physical Activities That Can Contribute To Mental Well-Being:

Aerobic Exercise:

- **Examples:** Running, Jogging, Brisk Walking, Cycling, Swimming, Dancing.

- **Benefits:** Aerobic Exercises Increase Blood Flow, Release Endorphins (The "Feel-Good" Hormones), And Contribute To Stress Reduction.

Strength Training:

- **Examples:** Weightlifting, Resistance Training, Bodyweight Exercises (E.G., Push-Ups, Squats).

- **Benefits:** Strength Training Not Only Enhances Physical Strength But Also Promotes Better Mood, Improved Sleep, And Increased Self-Esteem.

Yoga:

- **Examples:** Hatha, Vinyasa, Kundalini, Yin Yoga.
- **Benefits:** Yoga Combines Physical Postures With Mindfulness And Controlled Breathing, Promoting Relaxation, Stress Reduction, And Mental Clarity.

Pilates:

- **Examples:** Mat Exercises, Reformer Workouts.
- **Benefits:** Pilates Focuses On Core Strength, Flexibility, And Controlled Movements, Which Can Contribute To Improved Mood And Reduced Stress.

Tai Chi:

- **Benefits:** This Ancient Chinese Practice Combines Slow, Flowing Movements With Deep Breathing. It Is Known To Reduce Stress, Improve Balance, And Promote A Sense Of Calm.

Mindful Walking:

- **Benefits:** Taking A Walk While Paying Attention To Your Surroundings, Breathing, And Bodily Sensations Can Be A Mindful And Meditative Exercise, Promoting Relaxation.

Dance:

- **Examples:** Zumba, Ballet, Hip-Hop, Ballroom Dancing.
- **Benefits:** Dancing Is A Fun And Expressive Way To Improve Mood, Reduce Stress, And Increase Overall Well-Being.

Outdoor Activities:

- **Examples:** Hiking, Jogging In A Park, Biking Trails.
- **Benefits:** Spending Time Outdoors And Engaging In Activities Like Hiking Or Jogging In Natural Settings Can Have Positive Effects On Mood And Reduce Symptoms Of Depression.

Group Exercise Classes:

- **Examples:** Group Fitness Classes, Boot Camps, Spinning Classes.

- **Benefits:** Exercising In A Group Setting Can Provide Social Support, Motivation, And A Sense Of Community, Positively Impacting Mental Health.

Mind-Body Practices:

- **Examples:** Qigong, Feldenkrais Method, Alexander Technique.

- **Benefits:** These Practices Focus On The Connection Between The Mind And Body, Promoting Relaxation, Improved Posture, And Overall Mental Well-Being.

Sports:

- **Examples:** Soccer, Basketball, Tennis, Swimming.
- **Benefits:** Engaging In Sports Not Only Provides Physical Benefits But Also Fosters Teamwork, Social Interaction, And A Sense Of Accomplishment.

Interval Training:

- **Examples:** High-Intensity Interval Training (HIIT).
- **Benefits:** Short Bursts Of Intense Exercise Followed By Rest Periods Can Improve Mood, Boost Energy Levels, And Enhance Overall Fitness.

When Incorporating Physical Activity Into Your Routine For Mental Health, It's Essential To Choose Activities That You Enjoy And That Align With Your Fitness Level. Additionally, It's Advisable To Consult With Healthcare Professionals, Especially If You Have Existing Health Conditions Or Concerns. Regular Physical Activity, Combined With Other Self-Care Practices, Can Contribute Significantly To Maintaining And Improving Mental Well-Being.

Mindful Eating and Mental Health

Mindful Eating Is A Practice That Involves Paying Full Attention To The Sensory Experience Of Eating And Being Present In The Moment Without Judgment. This Approach To Eating Can Have Positive Effects On Mental Health In Several Ways:

• **Reduced Stress And Anxiety:** Mindful Eating Encourages Individuals To Focus On The Present Moment, Allowing Them To Let Go Of Worries And Anxieties Related To Past Or Future Events. This Can Contribute To A Reduction In Overall Stress Levels.

Improved Relationship With Food:

• Mindful Eating Promotes A Healthier Relationship With Food By Fostering Awareness Of Hunger And Fullness Cues. This Can Help Prevent Emotional Or Stress-Related Eating, Leading To More Balanced And Intentional Food Choices.

Enhanced Enjoyment Of Food:

• By Savoring Each Bite And Appreciating The Flavors, Textures, And Aromas Of Food, Mindful Eating Can Enhance The Overall Enjoyment Of Meals. This Positive Experience Can Contribute To Improved Mood.

Better Digestion:

• Mindful Eating Encourages Individuals To Eat More Slowly And Chew Their Food Thoroughly. This Can Aid Digestion And Prevent Issues Such As Indigestion Or Discomfort, Which May Impact Mental Well-Being.

Increased Awareness Of Emotional Eating Triggers:

• Mindful Eating Promotes Self-Awareness And Helps Individuals Recognize Emotional Triggers For Eating. Understanding The Connection Between Emotions And Eating Behaviors Can Support Better Emotional Regulation.

Prevention Of Overeating:

• By Paying Attention To Hunger And Fullness Signals, Individuals Are Less Likely To Overeat. This Can Contribute To Weight Management And Prevent Feelings Of Guilt Or Discomfort Associated With Overindulging.

Mind-Body Connection:

• Mindful Eating Emphasizes The Mind-Body Connection, Encouraging Individuals To Be In Tune With Their Bodies And Respond To Physical Hunger And Satiety Cues. This Awareness Can Extend Beyond Mealtime To Other Aspects Of Self-Care.

Reduced Binge Eating:

• For Individuals Prone To Binge Eating, Mindful Eating Can Be A Helpful Tool In Breaking The Cycle Of Impulsive And Emotional Eating. It Encourages A More Deliberate And Thoughtful Approach To Food Consumption.

Promotion Of Gratitude:

• Mindful Eating Encourages Individuals To Cultivate Gratitude For The Food They Have, Fostering A Positive Mindset And Appreciation For The Nourishment Provided By Meals.

Improved Body Image:

• By Promoting A Non-Judgmental Awareness Of The Eating Experience,

Mindful Eating Can Contribute To A More Positive Body Image And Reduced Self-Criticism Related To Food Choices.

• To Practice Mindful Eating, Individuals Can Focus On Aspects Such As Eating Slowly, Savoring Each Bite, Paying Attention To Hunger And Fullness Cues, And Minimizing Distractions During Meals.

It's Important To Note That Mindful Eating Is Not A Quick Fix But A Gradual And Ongoing Practice That Can Be Incorporated Into Daily Life. Combining Mindful Eating With Other Aspects Of A Healthy Lifestyle, Such As Regular Physical Activity And Balanced Nutrition, Can Contribute To

Overall Mental And Physical Well-Being. If Someone Has Concerns About Their Relationship With Food Or Mental Health, Seeking Guidance From Healthcare Professionals, Including Registered Dietitians And Mental Health Professionals, Is Advisable.

CHAPTER FIVE
Recipes for Schizophrenia-Friendly Meals

Creating Schizophrenia-Friendly Meals Involves Incorporating Nutrient-Dense Ingredients That Support Overall Mental Health And Well-Being. Here Are A Few Recipe Ideas That Focus On Balanced Nutrition And Include Ingredients Associated With Positive Mental Health:

Salmon and Quinoa Bowl:

Ingredients:

- Grilled or Baked Salmon Fillets
- Cooked Quinoa
- Steamed Broccoli And Carrots
- Sliced Avocado

- Lemon-Tahini Dressing (Mix Tahini, Lemon Juice, Garlic, And Olive Oil)

Instructions:

- Assemble Quinoa In Bowls, Top With Grilled Salmon, Steamed Vegetables, Avocado Slices, And Drizzle With Lemon-Tahini Dressing.

Vegetarian Stir-Fry:

Ingredients:

- Tofu Or Tempeh, Cubed
- Mixed Vegetables (Bell Peppers, Broccoli, Snap Peas)
- Brown Rice Or Quinoa
- Soy Sauce Or Tamari

- Garlic And Ginger, Minced

- Sesame Oil

Instructions:

- Stir-Fry Tofu Or Tempeh With Mixed Vegetables In Sesame Oil. Add Garlic And Ginger. Serve Over Brown Rice Or Quinoa, Drizzle With Soy Sauce Or Tamari.

Mango And Black Bean Salad:

Ingredients:

- Black Beans (Canned, Rinsed)

- Diced Mango

- Cherry Tomatoes, Halved

- Red Onion, Finely Chopped

- Cilantro, Chopped

- Lime Juice
- Olive Oil
- Salt And Pepper

Instructions:

• Mix Black Beans, Mango, Cherry Tomatoes, Red Onion, And Cilantro. Dress With Lime Juice, Olive Oil, Salt, And Pepper.

Chicken And Vegetable Curry:

Ingredients:

- Chicken Breast, Diced
- Mixed Vegetables (Zucchini, Bell Peppers, Carrots)
- Coconut Milk
- Curry Powder

- Turmeric, Cumin, And Coriander
- Garlic And Ginger, Minced
- Basmati Rice

Instructions:

• Sauté Chicken With Garlic And Ginger. Add Mixed Vegetables And Spices. Stir In Coconut Milk And Simmer Until Cooked. Serve Over Basmati Rice.

Greek Quinoa Salad:

Ingredients:

- Cooked Quinoa
- Cucumber, Diced
- Cherry Tomatoes, Halved
- Kalamata Olives, Sliced

- Feta Cheese, Crumbled

- Red Onion, Finely Chopped

- Olive Oil, Lemon Juice, Oregano

Instructions:

Combine Quinoa With Cucumber, Cherry Tomatoes, Olives, Feta, And Red Onion. Dress With Olive Oil, Lemon Juice, And Oregano.

Sweet Potato And Chickpea Buddha Bowl:

Ingredients:

- Roasted Sweet Potato Cubes

- Cooked Chickpeas

- Quinoa Or Brown Rice

- Spinach Or Kale

- Avocado Slices

- Tahini Dressing

Instructions:

• Assemble A Bowl With Roasted Sweet Potatoes, Chickpeas, Quinoa, Spinach Or Kale, And Avocado Slices. Drizzle With Tahini Dressing.

These Recipes Incorporate A Variety Of Nutrient-Dense Foods, Including Lean Proteins, Whole Grains, And Colorful Vegetables, Which Can Contribute To A Well-Rounded And Supportive Diet For Individuals Managing Schizophrenia. It's Essential To Consider Individual Preferences, Dietary Restrictions, And Consult With Healthcare Professionals For Personalized Advice.

Conclusion

Ultimately, The Management Of Schizophrenia Necessitates A Comprehensive Approach That Takes Into Account The Individual's Mental And Physical Health. Proper Nutrition Is Crucial For Individuals With Schizophrenia, And Working Together With Healthcare Specialists, Such As Dietitians And Nutritionists, Can Offer Tailored Advice.

• A Diet Suitable For Individuals With Schizophrenia Emphasizes The Consumption Of Foods That Are Rich In Nutrients, The Inclusion Of Well-Balanced Meals, And Taking Into Account Individual Preferences And Sensitivities. Omega-3 Fatty Acids,

Vitamins, And Minerals Are Essential For Maintaining Brain Function And Can Help Manage Symptoms.

• Aside From Nutritional Factors, Participating In Physical Activities That Enhance Mental Well-Being, Such As Aerobic Exercise, Resistance Training, And Mindfulness Techniques, Can Be Advantageous. Engaging In These Activities Helps To Alleviate Stress, Enhance Mood, And Promote Overall Mental Well-Being.

• Mindful Eating Is A Technique That Improves The Act Of Eating By Increasing Consciousness Of Food Selection, Appetite, And Satiety. It Has The Potential To Mitigate Emotional

Eating And Cultivate A More Wholesome Connection With Food.

• Collaborating With Healthcare Professionals, Such As Psychiatrists, Psychologists, And Nutritionists, Guarantees A Thorough And Unified Strategy For Managing Schizophrenia. The Partnership Between Mental Health And Nutrition Experts Enables The Development Of A Customized Strategy That Effectively Targets Both Mental Health Symptoms And Nutritional Requirements.

Integrating Dietary Modifications Into One's Daily Routine Requires Making Gradual Adaptations, Setting Achievable Objectives, And Making Conscious Decisions. It Is Crucial To

Commemorate Achievements, Maintain Adaptability, And Track Advancement When Striving For Total Well-Being.

To Effectively Manage Schizophrenia, It Is Crucial To Adopt A Comprehensive Approach That Includes Nutrition, Physical Activity, And Mental Health Assistance. By Adopting A Proactive And Cooperative Mindset, Individuals Can Improve Their Overall Quality Of Life And Well-Being.

THE END